The Heart Of A Hero: Daily Devotionals for Christian Paramedics

Delightful Devotionals

CONTENTS

Introduction

In the realm of emergency response, your calling goes beyond the sirens and flashing lights. As a paramedic, you stand on the front lines of compassion, as a beacon of hope in moments of crisis. This devotional journey is crafted specifically for you – the dedicated individual who carries the weight of others, often in the most challenging circumstances.

Each day, you navigate through the delicate balance of urgency and empathy, serving as a source of comfort and healing. This devotional is designed to uplift, inspire, and provide moments of reflection amidst the demanding nature of your noble profession. Within these pages, we embark on a journey to explore the intersection of your vital role and the timeless wisdom found in Scripture.

May this devotional be a companion in your moments of quiet reflection, a source of strength during challenging times, and a reminder of the profound impact you make in the lives of those you serve.

Your commitment to the call of service is truly a reflection of God's grace, and this journey is a testament to the extraordinary mission you fulfill every day.

Day 1: The Heart of Compassion

Verse of the Day:

Matthew 9:36 - "When he saw the crowds, he had compassion on them because they were harassed and helpless, like sheep without a shepherd."

Reflection:

In the demanding realm of paramedicine, where every call holds a story of urgency and vulnerability, let Matthew 9:36 be a guiding light. Picture the scene as Jesus looked upon the crowds, sensing their distress and recognizing their need for guidance.

In the same way, you, as a paramedic, are often met with individuals facing their most vulnerable moments. As you embark on this devotional journey, let the heart of compassion be the cornerstone of your service. Allow the empathy within you to echo the compassion that Jesus had for those in need. In moments of chaos and urgency, remember that your compassionate response holds the power to bring comfort and hope.

The weariness that can accompany the demanding nature of your profession finds peace in the compassionate care you provide. In the face of adversity, may your heart of compassion shine brightly, offering a beacon of hope to those you serve.

Journal:

1. Reflect on a specific instance in your paramedic career where compassion played a pivotal role in the care you provided. How did it impact both you and the person receiving care?

2. In challenging moments, how do you nurture and maintain a compassionate mindset to ensure the well-being of those under your care?

3. Consider the broader scope of your professional journey. How can you further cultivate and express compassion in your interactions with colleagues, patients, and their families?

Prayer:

Dear Lord, as I embark on this journey of reflection and devotion, I seek Your guidance to cultivate a heart of compassion. May the empathy within me mirror the compassion You demonstrated for the crowds. Grant me the strength to bring comfort and hope in the midst of chaos. In moments of weariness, may Your compassion sustain me, allowing me to serve with grace and kindness. Amen.

Day 2: Courage in Crisis

Verse of the Day:

Joshua 1:9 - "Have I not commanded you? Be strong and courageous. Do not be afraid; do not be discouraged, for the Lord your God will be with you wherever you go."

Reflection:

In the midst of crisis, where courage is required, let the words of Joshua 1:9 resonate in the core of your being. As a paramedic, you often find yourself on the frontlines, facing the unknown with unwavering courage.

The divine command to be strong and courageous is not a suggestion here but a resounding assurance that, in the midst of fear and uncertainty, you are not alone. The Lord your God is with you wherever you go.

Embrace each call, each challenging moment, with the strength that comes from knowing you are supported by a God who cares. Your courage is not just a response to the external crises you encounter but a reflection of the indomitable spirit within you.

It's a testament to your dedication to serving others, even when faced with adversity. Take heart, knowing that your courage is a beacon of hope for those who need it most.

Journal:

1. Recall a specific situation in your paramedic career where courage played a crucial role. How did your courage impact the outcome and what did you learn from that experience?

2. In moments of uncertainty, how do you draw upon your faith and the assurance that the Lord is with you? Reflect on a specific instance where this trust provided strength.

3. Consider the unique challenges you face in your profession. How can you cultivate and nurture courage as a consistent attribute in your personal and professional life?

Prayer:

Heavenly Father, in the face of crisis, I turn to Your command to be strong and courageous. Your presence is my assurance, and I find strength in knowing that You are with me wherever I go. Grant me the courage to face the unknown, to navigate challenges with resilience, and to be a source of hope for those in need. May Your guidance be my compass, and Your strength be my anchor. Amen.

Day 3: United in Service

Verse of the Day:

Ecclesiastes 4:9-10 - "Two are better than one because they have a good return for their labor: If either of them falls down, one can help the other up. But pity anyone who falls and has no one to help them up."

Reflection:

In the tapestry of paramedics, the bond between colleagues is a vital thread, woven with the strength described in Ecclesiastes 4:9-10. As you navigate the challenges of your calling, remember that the unity within your team multiplies the impact of your labor.

The scripture emphasizes the shared responsibility, mutual support, and the tangible benefits of collaboration. In the world of emergency response, the strength of your team is often the difference between adversity and triumph.

Take a moment to appreciate the interconnectedness among colleagues, recognizing that together, you form a resilient unit.

Lean on one another, for in unity, you find the strength to face the demanding nature of your profession. United in service, you become a powerful force for good, extending assistance not only to those you serve but also to each other in times of challenge.

Journal:

1. Reflect on a specific incident where the unity of your team made a significant impact on the outcome. How did collaboration enhance the quality of care provided?

2. Consider the dynamics within your team. How can you actively contribute to fostering a culture of unity and support among your colleagues?

3. Explore the idea of shared responsibility in your profession. In what ways can you strengthen your connections with fellow paramedics to ensure a more robust and unified response?

Prayer:

Gracious Lord, I thank You for the unity among colleagues, a source of strength in the paramedic journey. Help us to recognize the value of collaboration, to support and uplift one another in the face of challenges. May our shared labor be a testament to the power of unity, reflecting the interconnectedness You designed for us. Bless our teamwork, Lord, and guide us as we serve together. In Jesus' name, amen.

Day 4: Healing Hands: God's Instruments

Verse of the Day:

Luke 4:40 - "At sunset, the people brought to Jesus all who had various kinds of sickness, and laying his hands on each one, he healed them."

Reflection:

In your role as a paramedic, you embody the healing touch described in Luke 4:40. As the hands of Jesus brought peace to those in need, your hands become instruments of God's compassion and care. The scripture serves as a powerful reminder that healing is not just a physical process but a holistic act that encompasses the body, mind, and spirit.

Consider the impact of your hands in offering comfort, relief, and hope to those experiencing various forms of sickness. Your actions echo the divine healing witnessed in the Bible, illustrating the profound connection between faith and wellness.

In every patient encounter, may you recognize the sacred nature of your work, viewing your hands as extensions of God's grace and instrumen of restoration.

Journal:

1. Reflect on a specific instance where your actions, akin to layin hands, brought comfort and healing to someone in distress. Ho did this experience impact your perception of your role as paramedic?

2. Consider the holistic aspect of healing. How do you address n only the physical but also the emotional and spiritual well-bein of those under your care?

3. In challenging situations where healing seems distant, how ca you draw inspiration from the scripture to guide your actio and maintain a sense of purpose?

Prayer:

Heavenly Father, I am humbled by the opportunity to serve as a instrument of Your healing. May my hands carry the touch of You compassion, providing comfort and peace to those in need. Grant me th wisdom to approach each patient holistically, addressing not only the physical ailments but also their emotional and spiritual well-being. M Your healing power flow through me as I fulfill this sacred duty. Amen.

Day 5: Carrying the Weight of Others

Verse of the Day:

Galatians 6:2 - "Carry each other's burdens, and in this way, you will fulfill the law of Christ."

Reflection:

In the journey of being a paramedic, you are called to carry the burdens of others, embodying the spirit of Galatians 6:2. The scripture reminds us that by sharing the load, we fulfill the law of Christ – a profound directive that emphasizes empathy, compassion, and communal support.

As a paramedic, you often find yourself shouldering the weight of others' challenges, both physical and emotional. Acknowledge the significance of your role in alleviating burdens, recognizing that your service extends beyond the immediate moment of crisis. Every act of care, every compassionate response, contributes to fulfilling the higher calling of Christ's law.

In those instances where the weight feels heavy, remember that you are not alone, and by sharing the load, you exemplify the love and selflessness at the heart of your profession.

Journal:

1. Reflect on a specific experience where you felt the weight of someone else's burden during a call. How did this impact your understanding of your role as a paramedic?

2. Consider the emotional toll of your profession. How do you find ways to share the burdens with your colleagues or seek support when needed?

3. Explore practical ways to fulfill the law of Christ within your paramedic community. How can you actively contribute to creating a supportive environment for your colleagues?

Prayer:

Dear Lord, as I navigate the responsibilities of my role, I am mindful of the call to carry the burdens of others. Grant me the strength and compassion to fulfill this law of Christ, extending care beyond the immediate crisis. In moments of heaviness, may I find peace in Your presence and seek support from those who share this journey. Bless our collective efforts to lighten the burdens of those in need. Amen.

Day 6: Guidance in the Chaos

Verse of the Day:

Proverbs 3:5-6 - "Trust in the LORD with all your heart and lean not on your own understanding; in all your ways submit to him, and he will make your paths straight."

Reflection:

In the whirlwind of paramedic duties, the guidance of Proverbs 3:5-6 serves as a compass, steering you through chaos. The scripture implores you to trust in the Lord wholeheartedly, acknowledging that human understanding may falter in the face of complexity.

As a paramedic, you navigate unpredictable situations, for this reason, the assurance of divine guidance becomes your anchor. Embrace the wisdom of surrendering your ways to the Lord, seeking His guidance in every step. In the midst of chaos, trust that submitting to Him will bring clarity to your path.

Your role is not just a profession; it's a calling that requires reliance on God Himself. As you face the uncertainties, let the scripture be a source

of reassurance, guiding you through the complexities of your nobl
mission.

Journal:

1. Recall a challenging situation where you had to trust in th
   Lord's guidance. How did this reliance impact you
   decision-making and the overall outcome?

2. Reflect on moments of chaos in your profession. How can yo
   actively incorporate the guidance provided in Proverbs 3:5-6 int
   your daily practice?

3. Explore ways to deepen your trust in the Lord within the conte
   of your paramedic service. How can this trust influence you
   interactions with patients, colleagues, and the broade
   community?

Prayer:

Heavenly Father, in the midst of chaos, I turn to You for guidance. Hel
me trust in You with all my heart, leaning not on my own understandin
As I submit my ways to You, grant me clarity and wisdom to navigate th
complexities of my paramedic duties. May Your guidance be a constar
presence, leading me to serve with purpose and compassion. Amen.

Day 7: Patience in Urgency

Verse of the Day:

James 1:19 - "My dear brothers and sisters, take note of this: Everyone should be quick to listen, slow to speak, and slow to become angry."

Reflection:

In the urgency of your paramedic role, the counsel of James 1:19 becomes a guiding principle – to be quick to listen, slow to speak, and slow to become angry.

This scripture encapsulates the essence of patience, a virtue indispensable in the midst of emergencies. As you navigate urgent situations, embracing this wisdom can transform the dynamics of your interactions.

Patience in urgency is not merely a strategic approach but a reflection of empathy and understanding. Take a moment to listen attentively, allowing space for both verbal and non-verbal communication.

Let your responses be measured and your actions deliberate, recognizing the impact they may have on those in distress. In the whirlwind of urgency, your patience becomes a source of comfort and assurance.

Journal:

1. Reflect on a specific incident where practicing patience had a positive impact on the outcome of a call. How did your approach influence the dynamics of the situation?

2. Consider the challenges of maintaining patience in urgent scenarios. What strategies do you currently employ, and how can you further cultivate patience in your paramedic practice?

3. Explore ways to apply the principles of James 1:19 not only in emergency situations but also in your interactions with colleagues and the broader community.

Prayer:

Gracious Lord, grant me the patience needed to navigate the urgency of my paramedic duties. Help me to be quick to listen, slow to speak, and slow to become angry. May my actions reflect Your compassionate patience, bringing comfort and reassurance to those in need. Strengthen me to embody these virtues in the face of urgency. Amen.

Day 8: Hope in the Midst of Crisis

Verse of the Day:

Romans 15:13 - "May the God of hope fill you with all joy and peace as you trust in him, so that you may overflow with hope by the power of the Holy Spirit."

Reflection:

In the challenging landscape of crisis response, the promise of Romans 15:13 becomes a beacon of hope. As a paramedic, you navigate situations where hope can feel elusive, yet the scripture reminds you that the God of hope is present.

Trust becomes the key that unlocks the door to joy, peace, and an overflow of hope even in the darkest moments. Amidst the crises you face, cling to the assurance that God's hope is an unwavering anchor. Allow this hope to permeate your actions, infusing your responses with the transformative power of joy and peace.

Your role extends beyond the immediate physical needs; it encompasses the emotional and spiritual well-being of those you serve. May your presence radiate the hope described in Romans 15:13, bringing comfort and assurance to all those around you.

Journal:

1. Reflect on a specific crisis situation where the presence of hope made a significant difference. How did the assurance of hope influence your approach?

2. Consider ways to cultivate and maintain hope in your personal and professional life. How can you share this hope with colleagues and those under your care?

3. Explore the intersection of hope and trust in your paramedic journey. How does trusting in the God of hope impact your perspective during challenging times?

Prayer:

Heavenly Father, in the midst of crises, I seek the hope that only You can provide. Fill me with joy and peace as I trust in You, so that I may overflow with hope by the power of the Holy Spirit. May Your hope be a source of strength, comfort, and assurance in every situation I encounter. In Jesus' name, I pray, Amen.

Day 9: The Comforter in Trauma

Verse of the day:

Psalm 34:18 - "The Lord is close to the brokenhearted and saves those who are crushed in spirit."

Reflection:

In the midst of trauma, find peace in the comforting words of Psalm 34:18. As a paramedic, you often encounter individuals in their most vulnerable moments, and the assurance that the Lord is close to the brokenhearted serves as a foundation of hope.

Recognize that your presence becomes a conduit for God's comfort, a tangible expression of His closeness. Embrace the sacred responsibility of being a comforter in moments of trauma. Your actions echo the divine promise that the Lord saves those who are crushed in spirit. In your role, you become an instrument of God's compassion, offering comfort and support to those experiencing profound challenges.

May the scripture inspire you to approach each traumatic situation with a heart filled with empathy and the assurance of God's comforting presence.

Journal:

1. Reflect on a specific encounter where you witnessed the comfort of God in the midst of trauma. How did this experience shape your understanding of your role as a paramedic?

2. Consider the emotional impact of dealing with trauma regularly. How do you prioritize self-care to ensure you remain a source of comfort for others?

3. Explore practical ways to embody the closeness of the Lord in your interactions with trauma survivors. How can your presence bring comfort and healing to those in need?

Prayer:

Merciful Lord, in moments of trauma, I seek to be a vessel of Your comforting presence. Draw near to the brokenhearted through my actions, and grant me the wisdom to provide comfort to those crushed in spirit. May Your comforting love flow through me, bringing healing and hope to those I serve. In Jesus' name, Amen.

Day 10: Strength in Weariness

Verse of the Day:

Isaiah 40:31 - "But those who hope in the LORD will renew their strength. They will soar on wings like eagles; they will run and not grow weary, they will walk and not be faint."

Reflection:

In moments of weariness, find renewal and strength in the promise of Isaiah 40:31. As a paramedic, the demands of your role may leave you feeling exhausted, but this scripture offers a source of enduring strength.

Those who anchor their hope in the Lord will experience a revitalization that transcends physical weariness. Embrace the symbolism of soaring on wings like eagles, a powerful image of transcending challenges. Your hope in the Lord becomes the catalyst for endurance, allowing you to run without growing weary and walk without fainting.

Trust that, even in the midst of demanding situations, the divine promise of renewed strength will sustain you.

Journal:

1. Recall a time when you felt physically or emotionally weary in your role. How did you find strength to endure, and were there specific moments of renewal?

2. Explore the connection between hope in the Lord and your ability to persevere in challenging circumstances. How can this hope influence your approach to weariness?

3. Consider practical strategies to anchor your hope in the Lord for sustained strength. How can you integrate moments of spiritual renewal into your paramedic journey?

Prayer:

Heavenly Father, in moments of weariness, I turn to You for renewed strength. Help me to anchor my hope in You, trusting that I will soar on wings like eagles, run without growing weary, and walk without fainting. May Your promise of enduring strength be my source of resilience in the challenges I face. Amen.

Day 11: Balancing Compassion and Detachment

Verse of the Day:

Proverbs 11:17 - "Those who are kind benefit themselves, but the cruel bring ruin on themselves."

Reflection:

Striking a balance between compassion and detachment is a delicate art in the paramedic profession, and Proverbs 11:17 offers timeless wisdom.

The scripture highlights the profound impact of kindness, not only benefiting those you serve but also fostering personal well-being. Conversely, cruelty leads to ruin, emphasizing the importance of maintaining a compassionate heart.

As a paramedic, navigate the complexities of your role with a heart that reflects the kindness described in Proverbs. Recognize that your acts of compassion extend beyond immediate assistance; they contribute to your own well-being.

Balancing empathy with a level of detachment is crucial for maintaining emotional resilience, ensuring you can continue to provide quality care.

Journal:

1. Reflect on an experience where balancing compassion and detachment was challenging. How did you navigate this delicate equilibrium, and what lessons did you learn?

2. Consider the long-term effects of kindness in your paramedic interactions. How does practicing compassion contribute to your own well-being and the well-being of those around you?

3. Explore strategies to maintain emotional balance in your profession. How can you cultivate a compassionate heart while preserving the necessary level of detachment?

Prayer:

Gracious God, grant me the wisdom to balance compassion and detachment in my paramedic service. May my acts of kindness not only benefit those I serve but also contribute to my own well-being. Guard my heart against cruelty, and help me navigate the complexities of my role with a spirit of enduring kindness. Amen.

Day 12: Resilience in the Face of Tragedy

Verse of the Day:

Psalm 34:19 - "The righteous person may have many troubles, but the LORD delivers him from them all."

Reflection:

In the face of tragedy, draw strength from the assurance of Psalm 34:19. As a paramedic, you encounter the harsh realities of life, yet the promise in this scripture is a beacon of resilience.

Though troubles may be many, the Lord delivers the righteous from them all, providing a foundation of hope even in the darkest moments. Embrace the calling to righteousness, recognizing that your work as a paramedic is an avenue for delivering care in times of tragedy.

The resilience described in Psalm 34:19 is not merely personal; it's a shared journey where the Lord's deliverance becomes a source of hope and healing for those you serve.

Journal:

1. Reflect on a specific tragic incident where you witnesse resilience, either in yourself or in someone you were assistin; How did the Lord's deliverance manifest in that situation?

2. Explore the connection between righteousness and resilience i your paramedic service. How does living righteously contribu to your ability to navigate tragedies?

3. Consider ways to share the hope found in Psalm 34:19 wit colleagues and the broader community. How can the promise c deliverance be a source of encouragement in the face of tragedy?

Prayer:

Heavenly Father, in the face of tragedy, I seek Your deliverance and fin hope in the promise of Psalm 34:19. Grant me resilience as I navigate tr challenges of my paramedic service, and may Your deliverance be beacon of hope for those in distress. Amen.

Day 13: Teamwork in Crisis Response

Verse of the Day:

1 Corinthians 12:26 - "If one part suffers, every part suffers with it; if one part is honored, every part rejoices with it."

Reflection:

In the intricate dance of crisis response, embrace the wisdom of 1 Corinthians 12:26. As a paramedic, you are part of a dynamic team where each member's role is essential.

The scripture underscores the interconnectedness of the team; when one part suffers, the entire team feels it, and when one part is honored, there's shared rejoicing. Value the synergy within your team, recognizing that collaboration is vital in navigating crisis situations.

When challenges arise, remember that the shared burden lightens the load, and mutual support becomes a source of strength. Celebrate each success as a collective achievement, fostering a sense of camaraderie.

Journal

1. Reflect on a specific crisis response where teamwork played a crucial role. How did the interconnectedness of the team contribute to the overall success of the mission?

2. Consider the challenges of team dynamics in crisis situations. How can you actively contribute to fostering a sense of unity and mutual support within your paramedic team?

3. Explore ways to honor and celebrate the successes of your team. How can shared rejoicing strengthen the bond among team members?

Prayer:

Gracious God, in the intricate dance of crisis response, I acknowledge the importance of teamwork. Help me to appreciate the interconnectedness of my paramedic team, recognizing that when one suffers, we all suffer, and when one is honored, we all rejoice. May our collaboration be a source of strength and unity in the face of challenges. Amen.

Day 14: Self-Care for First Responders

Verse of the Day:

Matthew 11:28 - "Come to me, all you who are weary and burdened, and I will give you rest."

Reflection:

In the demanding role of a first responder, heed the compassionate call of Matthew 11:28.

As a paramedic, the weight of responsibilities can be overwhelming, but this scripture offers a divine invitation to find rest in the midst of weariness. Recognize the importance of self-care as a means to replenish your strength and rejuvenate your spirit.

Embrace the restorative power of coming to the Lord with your burdens. Prioritize self-care not as a luxury but as a necessary component of sustaining yourself in the demanding field of paramedicine.

In taking care of your well-being, you enhance your ability to provide effective and compassionate care to those you serve.

Journal:

1. Reflect on a time when the demands of your role as a first responder felt particularly burdensome. How did you find rest and rejuvenation in those moments?

2. Consider your current self-care practices. How can you align them with the invitation of Matthew 11:28 to come to the Lord for rest?

3. Explore proactive strategies to integrate self-care into your routine as a paramedic. How can prioritizing your well-being positively impact your ability to fulfill your responsibilities?

Prayer:

Loving Father, in the midst of the demanding role of a first responder, I come to You, seeking the rest You promise in Matthew 11:28. Grant me the wisdom to prioritize self-care, recognizing its importance in sustaining my well-being. May Your rest rejuvenate my spirit and empower me to provide compassionate care to those in need. Amen.

Day 15: Compassionate Communication

Verse of the Day:

Colossians 4:6 - "Let your conversation be always full of grace, seasoned with salt, so that you may know how to answer everyone."

Reflection:

In the realm of first response, embrace the guidance of Colossians 4:6, recognizing the power of compassionate communication. As a paramedic, your words carry weight in moments of crisis.

This scripture encourages conversations filled with grace, seasoned with the preserving quality of salt, creating an environment where answers are provided with wisdom and empathy. Consider the impact of your words on those you interact with, both colleagues and patients.

Strive for communication that reflects the grace described in Colossians, enhancing the overall experience for everyone involved. In moments of uncertainty, let your words be a source of comfort and reassurance.

Journal:

1. Reflect on a specific instance where communication played a crucial role in your paramedic duties. How did grace and empathy contribute to the outcome?

2. Consider your current communication style under pressure. How can you incorporate the qualities of grace and seasoned speech into your interactions with both colleagues and patients?

3. Explore ways to continually improve your compassionate communication skills. What steps can you take to enhance your ability to answer everyone with wisdom and empathy?

Prayer:

Gracious God, as a first responder, I seek Your guidance in fostering compassionate communication. May my conversations be filled with grace and seasoned with salt, reflecting the wisdom and empathy described in Colossians 4:6. Grant me the ability to provide answers that bring comfort and reassurance in moments of crisis. Amen.

Day 16: God's Guidance in Critical Decisions

Verse of the Day:

Proverbs 16:9 - "In their hearts humans plan their course, but the LORD establishes their steps."

Reflection:

Amid critical decisions, find peace in the assurance of Proverbs 16:9. As a paramedic, navigating complex situations requires careful planning, yet this scripture reminds you that the Lord ultimately establishes your steps.

Embrace the divine guidance that transcends human planning, trusting that your decisions are guided by a higher purpose. Recognize the significance of seeking the Lord's guidance in critical moments.

Allow Proverbs 16:9 to be a source of reassurance, acknowledging that your efforts are aligned with the divine order. In the face of uncertainty, trust that the steps you take are under the sovereign direction of the Lord.

Journal:

1. Reflect on a critical decision you had to make in your role as paramedic. How did seeking the Lord's guidance influence th outcome?

2. Consider the balance between human planning and divin guidance in your decision-making process. How can you ensur that your plans align with the steps the Lord establishes?

3. Explore ways to deepen your reliance on God's guidance i critical situations. What practices can you incorporate into you paramedic service to strengthen your connection with God?

Prayer:

Heavenly Father, in the midst of critical decisions, I turn to You guidance as described in Proverbs 16:9. Establish my steps, Lord, and le my decisions be in alignment with Your divine purpose. Grant m wisdom and discernment as I navigate complex situations, trusting tha Your guidance surpasses human planning. Amen.

Day 17: Endurance in Serving Others

Verse of the Day:

2 Timothy 4:7 - "I have fought the good fight, I have finished the race, I have kept the faith."

Reflection:

As a paramedic, choose today to draw strength from the endurance exemplified in 2 Timothy 4:7. Serving others in the field of emergency response can be a demanding race, and this scripture serves as a testament to finishing strong while keeping the faith intact.

Embrace the challenges with the assurance that your service is part of a noble fight. Reflect on the meaning of fighting the "good fight" in your paramedic role. Consider the ways in which you can endure with resilience, finishing each mission and keeping your faith unwavering.

May 2 Timothy 4:7 inspire you to persevere in serving others, knowing that your efforts contribute to the greater good.

Journal:

1. Reflect on a challenging moment in your paramedic service where endurance played a crucial role. How did you navigate the situation, and how did it impact your faith?

2. Consider the concept of the "good fight" in your role. What elements of your service align with fighting for the well-being of others?

3. Explore personal strategies for building endurance in your paramedic duties. How can you stay resilient while keeping your faith strong throughout your service?

Prayer:

Heavenly Father, grant me the endurance to fight the good fight in my role as a paramedic. As I navigate challenges and finish each mission, may I keep the faith unwavering. Inspire me to persevere in serving others, knowing that my efforts contribute to the greater good. In Jesus' name, I pray. Amen.

Day 18: God's Protection in Dangerous Situations

Verse of the Day:

Psalm 91:11 - "For he will command his angels concerning you to guard you in all your ways."

Reflection:

In the face of danger, find peace in the promise of Psalm 91:11. As a paramedic, your service often leads you into challenging and perilous situations. This scripture assures you that God's angels are commanded to guard and protect you in all your ways.

Trust in the divine protection that accompanies you in the line of duty. Reflect on the reassurance offered by Psalm 91:11, recognizing the presence of God's angels in your paramedic journey.

Whether responding to accidents, emergencies, or crises, rest in the knowledge that you are under the watchful care of heavenly guardians.

Allow this assurance to bring peace to your heart as you navigat
dangerous situations.

Journal:

1. Recall a specific instance in your paramedic service where you fe
    the protection of God in a dangerous situation. How did th
    experience impact your perspective on divine intervention?

2. Consider the challenges you face in dangerous situations. In wha
    ways does Psalm 91:11 provide comfort and assurance as yo
    fulfill your duties?

3. Reflect on practical ways to acknowledge and appreciate th
    protection of God's angels in your daily work as a paramedi
    How can you cultivate a sense of gratitude for the divir
    safeguard?

Prayer:

Heavenly Father, I place my trust in Your promise from Psalm 91:1
knowing that Your angels guard and protect me in all my ways as I serv
as a paramedic. Grant me courage in the face of danger and a dee
awareness of Your divine presence. May Your protection be a source c
comfort and assurance in every challenging situation. Amen.

Day 19: Empathy in Emotional Rescue

Verse of the Day:

Romans 12:15 - "Rejoice with those who rejoice; mourn with those who mourn."

Reflection:

In the realm of emotional rescue, embody the spirit of Romans 12:15. As a paramedic, you often find yourself providing care in moments of both joy and sorrow. This scripture encourages you to empathize with those you serve, rejoicing in their highs and mourning in their lows.

Cultivate a compassionate heart that mirrors the love and understanding of Jesus. Consider the significance of rejoicing and mourning alongside those in need. Romans 12:15 guides you to connect with the emotional experiences of others, fostering a sense of shared humanity.

In your role as a paramedic, let empathy be a guiding light, offering comfort and understanding to those undergoing emotional challenges.

Journal:

1. Reflect on a specific emotional rescue situation where you embraced empathy as a paramedic. How did Romans 12:15 influence your response?

2. Consider the importance of rejoicing and mourning with those in need. In what ways can you enhance your ability to connect emotionally with individuals during your rescue missions?

3. Explore ways to carry the spirit of Romans 12:15 into your daily interactions as a paramedic. How can empathy become a cornerstone of your compassionate care?

Prayer:

Gracious God, guide me to embody the empathy described in Romans 12:15 as I engage in emotional rescue situations. May I rejoice with those who rejoice and mourn with those who mourn, reflecting Your love and understanding. Grant me the strength to provide compassionate care in moments of both joy and sorrow. Amen.

Day 20: Grace Under Pressure

Verse of the Day:

Proverbs 14:29 - "Whoever is patient has great understanding, but one who is quick-tempered displays folly."

Reflection:

In moments of pressure, embody the wisdom of Proverbs 14:29. As a paramedic, exercising patience is a virtue that brings great understanding. This scripture reminds you that maintaining composure under pressure is a testament to your discernment.

Let patience be your guide, ensuring thoughtful and effective responses in challenging situations. Reflect on the value of patience as described in Proverbs 14:29. Recognize that, as a paramedic, your ability to remain composed influences the understanding and effectiveness of your service.

Embrace grace under pressure, knowing that patience is a powerful tool in navigating the complexities of your role.

Journal:

1. Recall a specific instance in your paramedic service when maintaining patience proved crucial under pressure. How did this experience impact the outcome?

2. Consider the relationship between patience and understanding in your role. How can you further cultivate patience to enhance your effectiveness in challenging situations?

3. Explore practical strategies for maintaining grace under pressure in your daily work as a paramedic. How can you incorporate patience into your response to various emergencies?

Prayer:

Heavenly Father, grant me the patience described in Proverbs 14:29 as I navigate the challenges of being a paramedic. May I maintain grace under pressure, allowing patience to guide my responses and actions. Strengthen my discernment and understanding in the moments that require composure. In Jesus' name, I pray. Amen.

Day 21: The Call to Serve: A Divine Assignment

Verse of the Day:

1 Peter 4:10 - "Each of you should use whatever gift you have received to serve others, as faithful stewards of God's grace in its various forms."

Reflection:

Embrace the divine assignment to serve, inspired by 1 Peter 4:10. As a paramedic, recognize that your skills and gifts are entrusted to you for the purpose of serving others.

This scripture encourages you to be a faithful steward of God's grace, using your unique abilities to bring comfort and healing to those in need. Reflect on the significance of viewing your role as a divine assignment.

1 Peter 4:10 reminds you that your service as a paramedic is not merely a profession but a calling, a way to express God's grace to those experiencing emergencies.

Approach each mission with a sense of purpose and commitment to being a faithful steward.

Journal:

1. Consider your unique gifts and skills as a paramedic. How does 1 Peter 4:10 inspire you to use these abilities as a form of God's grace in your service to others?

2. Reflect on the idea of being a faithful steward in your paramedic role. In what ways can you enhance your stewardship of God's grace throughout your daily interactions with patients and colleagues?

3. Explore how the concept of a divine assignment influences your perspective on the impact of your service. How can viewing your role through this lens bring a deeper sense of purpose and fulfillment?

Prayer:

Gracious God, thank You for entrusting me with the gifts and skills to serve as a paramedic. May I embrace the divine assignment described in 1 Peter 4:10, using my abilities as a faithful steward of Your grace. Guide me in bringing comfort and healing to those in need, fulfilling my calling with purpose and commitment. In Jesus' name, Amen.

Conclusion

As we conclude this devotional journey, I want to express my deepest gratitude for your unwavering dedication to the call of service. You, who stand at the crossroads of urgency and compassion, are a testament to the divine grace that flows through your every action.

In the moments of intense pressure, you've shown grace. In the face of uncertainty, you've embodied courage. Your hands, guided by skill and empathy, have become instruments of healing. This devotional sought to be a source of encouragement, a reminder of the profound impact your service makes, and a reflection of the divine purpose that threads through your noble calling.

As you continue to navigate the challenges and triumphs of being a paramedic, may the wisdom gleaned from these pages resonate in your heart. You are not just a responder to emergencies; you are a bearer of hope, a conduit of God's grace in its various forms.

May the verses, reflections, and prayers linger in your spirit, providing peace and inspiration.

And always remember that the echoes of your compassion reverberate far beyond the ambulance walls, leaving an indelible mark on those you've touched.

With a profound appreciation for your service and a prayer for your continued strength,

Delightful Devotionals